Nursing; a career with a Forever Future

A Practical Guide to Nursing school

BY WILLIE J. FORD

Order this book online at www.trafford.com
or email orders@trafford.com

Most Trafford titles are also available at major online book retailers.

Printed in the United States of America.

ISBN: 978-1-4269-1734-9 (sc)

*Our mission is to efficiently provide the world's finest, most comprehensive book
publishing service, enabling every author to experience success. To find out how to
publish your book, your way, and have it available worldwide, visit us online at
www.trafford.com*

Trafford rev. 09/22/2010

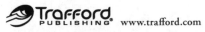 www.trafford.com

North America & international
toll-free: 1 888 232 4444 (USA & Canada)
phone: 250 383 6864 ♦ fax: 812 355 4082

DEDICATION

This book is dedicated to two fine nurses who have gone before you. Lillie Ross, my loving mother who encouraged and inspired me and my dear mother in law Dolores King who continues to support me.

FOREWARD

Kathryn Ryan RN, BSN, MSA Clinical Educator
Milwaukee VA Medical Center

In an easy to read format, Willie Ford writes about the process involved to enter a nursing program. As the reader you feel like you are having a personal conversation with Willie as he shares some of his personal experiences on the road to becoming a nursing professional. He takes you on journey by guiding you through the processes involved to enter a nursing program. He is honest about how this the commitment will affect your personal life and responsibilities.

Once in the nursing program Willie advises you on both human and material resources that will help you to succeed. However he frequently cites that you are ultimately responsible for your own success.

In Willie's writing there are threads of the challenges in nursing that you will face as a student and as a professional nurse. He presents this information not to discourage, but rather to demonstrate the need to be flexible and adaptable to a variety of situations always putting the patient at the center of care.

I especially liked the inspirational stories of the two women at the end of the book. Their life journeys give us hope, courage and strength to persevere toward achieving our goals. The rewards of nursing are often more than monetary!

What are you waiting for…start reading!

CONTENTS

10 CHARASTERISTICS OF THE SUCCESSFUL NURSING STUDENT

When asked the question of what would she look for in the successful nursing student noted author, speaker and educator, Laurie Materna, Phd, RN, who currently utilizes her skills as a nursing instructor drew up a specific list of the qualities or characteristics she would most like to see her students bring to the nursing program or develop under the auspices of its instructors.

1. Ability to draw upon theoretical and personal knowledge base when exploring new issues.

2. An inquiring mind, understanding how to ask questions and how to probe deeper for details.

3. Ability to accurately assess own learning needs and to challenge self to learn more.

4. Possess humanistic interpersonal skills and ability to communicate therapeutically (caring, respect, compassion, empathy).

5. Ability to organize self and manage time to effectively prioritize nursing cares, and the ability to explain rationale for prioritization.

6. Willing to collaborate with ancillary health care team to promote positive client outcomes.

7. Ability to identify teaching needs and demonstrate patient-centered teaching approach for patient/family.

8. Ability to identify and utilize unit and community resources to promote positive patient outcomes.

9. Demonstrate ability to delegate cares and supervise Para-professional staff while behaving as a role model for nursing.

10. Being an independent, flexible, creative, out-of-the-box thinker who work through and problem-solve issues/concerns.

Nursing instructor Materna is the author of two books encompassing learning and its educational aspects for adults. They are two of the Jump start series, Jump Start the Adult Learner: How to Engage and Motivate Adults Using Brain Compatible Strategies and Jump Start the Adult Learner: Smarter Strategies for Better Teaching. She is currently teaching at the Milwaukee Area Technical College located in Milwaukee Wisconsin.

Within the next five years as the current crop of nurses enter into their retirement years (the baby boomers), this country will need an average of 10,000 new nurses a week for four years just to replace them. Even that will not keep up with the demand imposed by the now nurse starved health care system. This book is dedicated to those tireless souls who have and are soon to dedicate their lives and spirits to the preservation and practice of the nursing profession. A livelihood that will take them to the forefront of the health care system in the modern world.

With the decrease in production jobs in the United States and an increase in the service sector more and more students are gravitating toward the nursing profession as a means of a challenging, rewarding and financially secure future for themselves and their families.

Even more of today's nursing students are looking for that magic bullet or formula that will make studying much easier and comprehension more attainable. There are experts who address such topics and one being nursing instructor Materna who we spoke of earlier. One word she has lived in her life's work is a word I am sure you have heard much about. That single word is dedication, that single act of devoting oneself to achievement in the nursing field.

From now on the act of studying will as some of you might know take on different forms not unlike that of high school or even some college classes you may have taken. Nursing classes as you have probably heard are definitely different; they take on a life of their own because they deal in the well being and precious health of at risk patients.

In interviewing a Vietnam veteran who at the time was an established nursing student, he shared how nursing school and nursing instructors particularly unnerved him more than combat. They're not quite the same but it was a point well taken. Regardless, classes, exams and study techniques are tough and as well they should be. Hopefully, the tips in this book will be useful to you and have a place in your study connection.

Alright, now that you're ready to take your first several steps as a nursing student to new heights, we will not waste your time. There are many nursing instructors and future patients awaiting you.

A while ago when we were children and we were just starting our academic career most of us didn't feel that we had any choice in attending school. Most of us chose to follow the group and attend to our studies while a few of us never did get it. Those never did the assigned homework and never studied for test. They dropped out of school and with some that was seen as a badge of honor at the time. Today many of those are returning to school and those who are changing careers for what ever reason are choosing to find their way back to classes and are choosing nursing as a career choice.

ENTRANCE EXAM

Unless you're graduating from college and are entering nursing school you will find that you need to take an entrance exam to qualify. This determines for the school if you are capable of completing the course as offered. Subjects covered in this exam are multiple math problems along with those of reading and English comprehension.

WHO DECIDES WHO MAKES A GOOD NURSE

That's a good question. The answer is it's you who decides who will make a good nurse. Everyone carries around a mental image of what a nurse should look like. The people who made that decision were the same ones who said that all construction workers should be a certain type of male. We now know that not to be true, it was that double edge sword tradition along with the sugar coated social trends invented by Hollywood as they made the rules in the casting office over coffee and brandy. Some instructors had been so brainwashed and protective of their own livelihood that they thought of themselves as gatekeepers posted there to see that only those who fitted their ideal nursing image should pass. That is not the case now; their successors want to see the best qualified students succeed no matter what gender, age or color.

ABANDON HOPE ALL YE WHO ENTER HERE

This is the inscription at the gates of hell from Dante's Divine Comedy. No, nursing school is not the equivalent of hell but I'm sure it is just as anxiety producing and as well it should be. It's a reminder to us from the pit of our stomach to the splitting headache that we are in the middle of a serious phase in our educational life and it deserves our utmost attention, respect and serious preparation.

PRE REQUISITES

Yes, you need the pre classes if you have not had them before or as they are called your pre requisites. Those are the general science classes and the math classes you will need. Don't let the word math scare you. My belief is that if you can count money you can make it in your math classes. Don't let anyone tell you any differently; don't ever let anyone tell you that you can't pass the math classes. There are tutors available to supplement your classes. There are other general education classes that may be required by the school such as English or economics prior to entering the program. This would depend on where you are in your academic life. A school counselor will be happy to investigate and alert you to any and all classes you need and changes you need to make. Although the counselors are an important resource don't let them dictate your every move. I know a woman whose counselor told her she couldn't possibly take two science classes at the same time it would just be too hard. This woman not wanting to wait an extra semester to get into clinicals decided to take both classes anyway. She passed both science classes and the other classes she was taking and maintained her honor student status. To be fair to the counselor in his experiences most people would have failed at this endeavor. It's important that you keep your own capabilities and limitations in mind. She knew she could handle it so she went for it. If you're working and have three kids be realistic. And remember taking a class over is expensive. Don't set yourself up for failure if you are in a hurry. Keep in mind you are in charge of yourself and your destiny.

Willie J. Ford

Counselors are a good resource but they haven't been through the course. Also talk to other students who are already in the program, instructors or recent graduates. After you've taken all of your pre requisites and lived through the waiting list. Don't let a five year waiting list scare you off. Some of the people who are ahead of you on the list will drop off for various reasons; they couldn't complete prerequisites, changed their mind, or someone ahead of them already in the program failed a clinical rotation (scary thought isn't it?).

In most cases you will be required to have a physical exam and updated vaccinations. In some cases the hepatitis B vaccination is optional. I strongly recommend getting this vaccination. Even if you are very careful it's most likely that at some point you will be exposed to another persons blood.

Then, hopefully you have your CPR class well behind you. CPR classes can be taken with the Red Cross or schedule classes at your college. They can also be taken in your community such as the YMCA and church programs. Either way you will need it to participate as a student nurse in training. You will not, I repeat you will not be allowed to participate in your nursing classes without it. Such certificates can be renewed every two years or every year depending on what is required by the school. Be sure and check, there is more than one type of CPR certification. Other needful things are all of the required books, pamphlets and supplies which we will go into more details as we go through this manual. Then congratulations, you are ready to suspend your real life and become a nursing student.

WANT TO BE A NURSE?

Of course some of us have different situations none of which are exactly the same. We all have different life circumstances and we need different things to survive this world. We all want love, respect, understanding friends and obedient children but that's not everyone's reality. There are single mothers and there are married mothers There are those of us who will make our opportunities, those of us who refuse an opportunity and there are those of us who humbly ask for an opportunity. Some nursing students have even been known to be homeless at times while others have felt that they had the weight of the whole world on their shoulders. Anyone of us can become a nurse and anyone of us can dedicate ourselves to the hard work that is needed. As in anything some of us find that going through life seems a little easier for others. Many people have made it through nursing school, young people, grandmothers, former bankers, you name it. The diversity you find in nursing schools today is endless. Caution, if you are a convicted felon or have any kind of drug related charges in your past you are not likely to get accepted into school and are less likely to be granted a license. If you have any doubts about passing a background check you might want to talk to an advisor before spending money on any classes. You should seriously consider another line of work for your own peace of mind. Imagine how it was with a student who was not allowed to graduate because of a records check (more will be discussed on this subject later in this pamphlet).

Willie J. Ford

FINDING THE TIME FOR NURSING SCHOOL

Time is your friend and you need to manage your friend wisely. You might not think so but remember there is life after nursing school and there is a light at the end of the tunnel.

The first thing you need to know is that despite the problems of the economy there is some help available. Student loans can be counted on through the Financial Aid office of your school or university provided you qualify. Searching out other student loans from family members including parents may be one of the alternate sources you can count on. Besides paying for classes you may need it for living funds. If you don't have a wife, husband or some other loved one to help you make ends meet. You may need a part time job or sadly as the case may be for other people, two part time jobs, so utilize your support system. If child care is needed talk to your counselors at school, your family members and your most trusted friends. Remember your success will depend on them as well as yourself. To reiterate talk to your counselors, they get paid to answer your questions; they get paid to help you. If need be and one is available, they will help you to find a job. Remember, they cannot justify their existence without you, the student. Among other things, they assist you in arranging your classes; they are your number one resource. There are also the employers at health facilities that offer programs that will pay for your nursing classes. Through reimbursing you or outright paying for any classes or fees you incur, stipulating that you work for them for a certain number of years after you graduate.

WAITING LIST

We mentioned before the dreaded waiting list of nursing school. Not everyone who wants to go to nursing school can get in right away. They operate on a first come first served basis or by lottery. When more students sign up for classes than there are spaces for the remainder are put on a waiting list. Now don't be discouraged by the name waiting list because it usually moves pretty fast depending on how many people want to sign up. It will move about as fast as a waiting list can move considering people change their minds. Some potential students move out of town or get sick and drop out of contention for a slot. For whatever the reasons they all have more pressing problems that make it impossible for them to continue. This is where your perseverance pays off; it will continue to move you up in the list until you're called. Which could be faster then you expect so be ready.

WHERE DOES YOUR NURSING SCHOOL GET ITS ACCREDITATION?

One thing you should be interested in is the accreditation of your chosen nursing school. It is your right and your obligation to assess what type of accreditation your school holds. This is the standard in which the schools themselves are held to and graded.

The type of accreditation states that your schools curriculum has been reviewed and has been found to be acceptable to their organization. Different accreditation has been assign to different nursing programs. The largest of these organizations located in the United States are the National League of Nursing Accrediting Commission (NLNAC) and The Commission on Collegiate Nursing Education(CCNE). NLNAC accredits associates, bachelors and masters degree programs and CCNE will only accredit bachelor and masters degrees. Your potential school will be happy to give you the name of the organization who has given them their accreditation. Remember there are different levels of accreditation and being aware of how your nursing education is viewed by nursing organizations will be very important to you when you are ready to start your nursing career. Accreditation also reveals to you what locals and what states would recognize your license to practice.

THE ACCEPTANCE LETTER

Your first order of business will began when you receive your acceptance letter into nursing school. It will be very cordial and of course business like as it tells you the time and place to report for your first orientation. You will consider it some of the best news you will ever receive, your heart will pound as you realize that your life is finally moving into another phase. Your first obligation on receiving your notice is to gather up your required supplies (we will delve more into this later) and make any arrangements needed to free up time to attend your classes.

MEETING YOUR NURSING INSTRUCTOR

Meet your new role model, your new boss, your new friend and your new confidant. Well, I might have gone a little overboard with that phrase but I want you to get the message. During your first orientation lecture you will get your first chance at meeting your instructor. This will be your chance to meet and greet and stand by bewildered as everyone rushes by you to get a good seat in the lecture hall. There will be several nursing instructors depending on how large your class is. Only one will have your name on his or her list. This large class will be divided into numerical groups with each instructor taking a group. The purpose of each group having its own instructor assures that more students will survive the coming semester.

Classes at times will breed frustrations with your instructor, do not, I repeat do not let anger get the better of you. Do not challenge this person and I state person because your instructor does not necessarily have to be a woman. Men do make and are excellent nursing instructors as well. Do not pretend that you know more than her/him, they are the instructor and do not argue with them because it is virtually impossible to convert them to your way of thinking.

If you believe that they made a mistake on an issue address it in an adult manner. Do not attempt to humiliate them but treat them as you would your boss because in a manner of speaking they are. Rudeness has no place in this profession or you will dig a hole for yourself that could be difficult to later climb out of. Do not make personality an issue, she is there to teach and guide you through the nursing process. It is really imperative that you don't question her teaching skills just to make yourself look smarter. Any legitimate concerns you may have she should address those; she is after all a representative of the school.

Don't let rumors about certain instructors being "tough" worry you. Sometimes instructors that challenge you give you your best educational opportunities. You don't want to glide through nursing school having the most laid back instructors who give you light patient loads. You won't be prepared for the real world.

SETTING CLASS SCHEDULES

Classes are generally like crowds because given time they too will tend to thin out. During the beginning of the semester nursing classes can average anywhere between 50 to 70 or more students, sometimes more sometimes less given the number of students assigned to the class. While this was mentioned earlier it should be noted again that the larger class is divided into smaller groups each with its own nursing instructor at the head of these groups. The smaller class schedules can then be divided into three large sections Lecture/ Study groups and Clinicals with different days set aside for each. For the sake of designations Lectures are when the full class of students are gathered in an auditorium or large lecture room to hear a designated instructor give a lecture on the weeks study subject. Then the full class is expected to re-form into their smaller class with their individual instructor to study and discuss the presented subject. Every week on lecture day the curriculum is adhered to as the study of practical knowledge. The reading of text books and the taking of test, quizzes and various smaller lectures on what will be covered in said test.

Labs are on the days in which the instructors in the same class present the studies on different nursing techniques. These demonstrations can cover anything from the selection of bathing a baby to doing bladder irrigations depending on where the class is in its curriculum. Which as the semester moves on, clinicals are on the days in which the class puts into practice those techniques in hospitals or nursing homes depending on whichever you are assigned to at the time. This is called a Rotation, alternating from one care facility to another. Learning to function in the different environments and the abilities needed to safely develop in each.

MEETING YOUR NEW CLASSMATES

Meeting new nursing classmates is a lot like the adventures of speed dating. First you meet very quickly during the first orientation; hopefully you will meet a few you will like because you will be spending a lot of time with them. Your bonding time will start during the first lecture then it's off to the races. Time literally speeds up around you and there is a lot to cover. Which means you as a student must reset your internal clock to correspond with your classes otherwise you will be left behind. There is a huge amount of information to cover and you will often wonder how you will be able to do it. If the campus is unfamiliar to you, you will be off to find your way around, to the bookstore, to get a locker (a word of advice, keep two lockers) to find and qualify for parking. Hopefully you will be able to find adequate parking on or near campus. Continuing this leisurely pace you should tour the campus and familiarize yourself with where the auditorium and other lecture sites are located. Arranging some of these tours with classmates who you will study and train with will afford you a tremendous opportunity to make lifelong friends who will remain in the profession thereby offering a support system unsurpassed in other professions.

PART TIME JOB/PART TIME SCHOOL

Not everyone can go to school while their parents pay the bills, although it would be nice most of us aren't able to qualify. I can't sit here and tell you what your situation is, only you know that and better than anyone else. Only you will be able to find the perfect balance of school and work, it won't be easy. It's a lot like life, it's full of questions. Will you have to take one class a semester and work the majority of your hours or vice versa? You will be allowed to make your variations on the two; it is possible, it has been done. It will just set your graduation back a bit.,,,,,,,,,,,,,,,,,,,,,, NOTE to your counselor.

STUDY GROUPS FACT OR FICTION

Nursing students like any other students are always looking for an edge in studying, mainly because the classes are so intensive. These classes are designed to move the students quickly through the program to gain the knowledge to successfully complete the course. One way of studying, that students gravitate towards is the age old concept of group studying. A study group despite its name can consists of anywhere from two to twenty students or more. This would make it a democratically structured class without an instructor, needing the input and ideas from each member. Depending on the number they arrive at that would allow them to effectively exchange those ideas and promote interesting discussions pertaining to the subjects at hand. The study group, to be successful must depend on the participation of again, all of its members lest the group degenerates into a purely social gathering. The group studies potential questions and answers and offers suggestions on what the next test may cover. The group also communicates with classes that covered the same exams before them always searching for clues of what to expect in their next test.

WHEN IT IS OK TO SLEEP IN CLASS

At some point in your studious life you may literally wake up to find that you had been sleeping during a lecture or demonstration in a class. Don't panic; don't attempt to push the replay button. You may even wonder why no one woke you during the good part. The instructor may not even wake you; every college student that studies hard knows that sleep comes when you can get it. We're all adults here and you are no longer in high school, no ones going to write a note to your mom. The repercussions for not studying are well known and if you don't want to participate then you're wasting your money which would be punishment enough. If for some good reason or not so good reason you are somewhat incapacitated or late for class or feel that you didn't particularly pay attention to lecture.

Have your self a backup plan, someone who can take good notes and are willing to share them with you but just remember that someday you may have to return the favor.

PICKING A CLINICAL SITE

TA! DA!!!, holy moly, they have the list of clinical sites up on the board and in reality you may have a good number of them to choose from. Between five and eight hospitals and nursing homes and different wards, pre and post surgical along with long term care. In choosing the site for your clinical you may want to base your choices on simple reasons. If you particularly like the instructor and if you have heard that she is tough and unyielding. Maybe you are intrigued by how far it is from your place of residence or school. Could it be that this clinical will be Maternal nursing and you just love babies. Hey, I know your best friend and you can be in the same clinical together and you just know that you have a great chance to pass if you study together. Whatever the reason you choose, here is another reason to consider maybe, just maybe you would like to work there when you graduate. Many clinical sites use teaching as a recruitment tool to attract excellent students who eventually become excellent employees.

WHEN STUDENTS ARE ELIMINATED FROM THE PROGRAM

Thus begins the practice of eliminations from the nursing program, which some of the causes can be rooted in the failure of too many written exams and the inability to maintain a passing average. This could mean failing at any point deemed unacceptable and being dropped from the class. Elimination could also occur during a clinical at the local hospital or nursing home. It could be while performing various treatments and/or the dispensing of medication by the students that they are found to be unsafe or inadequate by the instructor. In which case the Instructor waits until the end of the clinical day or right on the spot (in privacy of course) dismisses the offending student nurse from the remainder of the program.

MAKING THE COMEBACK

If for some reason you find that you and the nursing program you have chosen are not compatible and you were asked by the Instructor to sit out the remainder of the semester. Could it be that it is believed by your Instructor that you do not comprehend the material as it is intended by the program developers? Perhaps there is another problem such as your test taking average is too low to continue in the program. Maybe just maybe you are seen by your Instructor as being just too eager to overdose your patients on their scheduled pain medication. Another reason is that at the time, you are seen as a walking, talking, and breathing medical hazard. There are other alternatives; you may choose to explore your options to enter into discussions with the Deans representatives to realize any choices they may have to offer. Other ways are to utilize tutors who may be staffing the Nurses Lab and are to there to strengthen any weaknesses you feel that you may need help in. Most accredited schools do offer such programs; you just need to be aware of just what their program has on the books. Should the time come, and it may not, that you are dropped from a nursing program, you do have a second a third, or even a fourth, fifth and sixth chance. Usually, and I am not exaggerating, the second time is really a charm.

THE GREAT COMEBACK KID

So what happens should the unthinkable happen? No, I don't mean your uncle Joe with his wife and his eight undisciplined kids come to live with you. I mean that if you are dropped from the program after all of your hard work and money borrowed. There is a fail safe to that problem. You won't be the first student to take that plunge or the last. It has been a sad reality to other aspiring nurses and they have on more occasions landed on their feet as you will.

As we have stated before nursing classes run in rotation, meaning for example should you decide to discontinue or are forced out against your will or just decide to take a breather, you should be able to rotate back into another spot on the roster. This is how it would work, should you flunk out on your participation in say the middle of Maternity rotation (birthing them babies).Then you would have to sit out the rest of that session and the following classes until the maternity class comes around again probably in the next semester. That little setback would make you unable to graduate with the current class you started with. Using your idle time wisely you would be studying to correct your last rotations mistakes. Then you would be eligible to start again at the beginning of the same class you were dropped from, hence the rotation.

What if you decide that you are just as fed up with your current nursing school as it is with you. Maybe, for some reason only you can see is that the Instructor just doesn't like you. Much as we like to think otherwise personalities can clash. The next best thing you can do is to search for a school or college or as the name implies a university that is much more suitable to your learning abilities, your personality, and your educational funds or perhaps closer to home. Whatever your reasons let them be realistic. Do a fair self assessment of your abilities and discuss them with your pending nursing school. Then satisfy all of the entry requirements for a transfer. Remember that if you are collecting student loans they will add up if you fail to graduate on time with your class. Your lender will expect repayment whether you graduate or not. Repayment is usually asked for approximately a year after you graduate, sooner if you drop out.

STRESSED OUT

Nursing school unlike most training schools produce a stressful environment all of their own. Classes move so fast and there is so much to absorb in such a short time that many people can't keep up. Stress bleeds out into your social and family life as well. For the serious older student who has to juggle children and a complete relationship along with the monetary problems that tend to go along with it. Dealing with school and an ill relationship can at times be quite depressing.

If your relationship is already on shaky ground, nursing school can be the thing that will drive it over the edge.

This manual will be honest with you in all aspects of this subject. On scheduling your time between studying and family life, remember you need understanding backup and support from your husband/boyfriend/wife girlfriend/children and other family members, even your boss should you have to work. Lovers and family members can sometimes become outrageously jealous of the time your homework and classes take away from them. Please continue to explain to them that this is only temporary at the time and do attempt to designate some time to spend with them, treat your self to a break with them when possible. Use your down time from school wisely whether picking up extra time to work or extra time to spend with family, friends and loved ones .It will all come back to you in a positive manner. If you let it life can almost become a nightmare but many people have done it and have survived to tell the tale. Looking back on your experiences after you have earned a nursing degree, you could well find that it was some of the most enjoyable times of your life.

BACKGROUND CHECK

We did mention this earlier but I believe that this is a touchy subject and needs to be delved into a little deeper for your and my sake. I want to give you the lowdown thorns and all as I see it. Nursing is one of the professions that legally dispenses and has contact with numerous drugs designated as control substances. Morphine pills, morphine patches, Oxycontin and all of the other so called candy that gets little people in such big trouble. Nurses are just like other people, they can fall into that trap as well.

Once the pre nursing student is accepted for enrollment in the nursing program their life's history with the legal system is open for review. Just as when seeking employment or permission to work anywhere there is a chance to work with vulnerable people or substances that can be used to support an illegal trade a background check is done. A response is not always instantaneous due to the demand of employers and law enforcement agencies for such information. There have been instances where the student has successfully passed the nursing program only later to be refused graduation as a nurse but allowed to switch majors to become employable. Another time the graduated nursing student was refused employment due to the sensitive gray areas in the dealing in illegal drugs. Even as with other professions undesirables do seep through. These problems are overseen by the nursing board and they do control the licenses of its nursing professionals. Using their powers of suspending and revoking such licenses as needed.

ATTENDANCE

Absenteeism will not be tolerated and chronic absences will especially not be tolerated. If you miss a little you miss a lot and it may be difficult or even impossible to keep up. Where there is an illness of a child, a death in the family or family trouble or an illness to yourself. If you believe that you will not be able to keep up your attendance then see it as a fore warning.

As mentioned before and it cannot be stressed enough, if one or more of these problems plague you and you feel overwhelmed. If you feel that you can't continue use your noggin and voluntarily separate from the nursing program. You can always re-enter on your own terms during the next rotation or the next year. If you decide to drop out please remember to not give up on your dreams.

SURPRISE

This book just begs for an unscientific scientific survey and not wanting to disappoint, here goes. Several nursing school students and graduated nurses were asked a question. They were promised anonymity.

What surprised you most about nursing school?

ANSWERS:

#1 … "Clinicals surprised me the most; I had a hard time dealing with the dignity issues of the patients."

#2 … "All of the information we were expected to absorb at one time."

#3 … "How many people failed in my rotation."

#4 … "That it was going to be so hard."

#5 … The politics that men can't make good nurses."

#6 … "Seeing a baby born."

#7 … "I felt isolated in clinicals from the regular nursing staff."

#8 … "The attitude of the Instructors, they were so critical of the students."

#9 … "The enormous amount of reading."

#10 … "How fast and rigorous the nursing program was."

#11 … "The amount of study."

#12 … "Studying anatomy with dead bodies."

#13 … "The high standards."

As you can see, beginning nursing school can impact different students in different ways. Leaving all feeling somewhat figuratively bruised and battered but never the less feeling a great deal of accomplishment. The medical world offers a cultural shock to the uninitiated, which will soon wear off as the blushing recedes.

LEADERSHIP

Nursing schools look for leadership in their students not only being a leader but showing others how to lead as well. This means that what any good leader would do is take responsibility for their charges. "You are expected to be nice but not too nice" as one Instructor was heard to say. She also responded when asked what is "too nice?" She was "nice" enough to explain that "A nurse has to be assertive to the point of advocating for the patient. This would tend to mean that your patient is in your care and the patient depends on your care. Your tour is to be built around your care for your patient."

There is a point that a student should strive for during your tour of caring for your patient. See that all of your patients that are dependent on you are taken care of, don't leave anything undone and expect someone to take care of it for you. If that means that on occasions you will miss lunch or break then so be it. Should you survive to work clinicals in a nursing home or a hospital you will most likely be asked to supervise CNA's. They are deserving of your respect and it's highly possible you will have worked as a CNA or you will. Then you probably know that they are the eyes and ears of the nurse so be professional and they will help you make it through clinicals safely. Keep on your toes, this subject will be repeated again elsewhere in this manual.

STUDENT TOOLS

The tools at a students disposal can run the gamut from book bags to patches, so with the space here allotted to me I will try to name a few. Number one, you will be required to purchase a school nursing uniform. It will have to be in a school designated color. Now you may believe you can purchase those uniform colors anywhere. That may not be necessarily true, your school may have a contract with a special uniform store or they may be selling them in their store. Expect to pay more then you would stopping at the local ABCD department store but remember after you graduate you can still get a little wear out of it. You will just need to take the nursing school patch off the shoulder. Which brings up the subject of the nursing school patch, you will need to purchase two of these. One patch for your school uniform and a second one just in case. You will need a stethoscope for training on your patients and hopefully you won't need to buy the top of the line. Just wrap it around your neck and you look like a nurse already. It's handy for taking blood pressures along with heart and lung assessments.

Forms, forms and more forms for you to fill out and just to name a few you will need practice in are Admission forms, Pain assessments, Full body assessments and Discharge assessments , just to name a few.

DO'S AND DONT'S OF CLINICALS

#1.. DO get plenty of sleep the night before.

#2. Do be prepared for your clinicals.

#3. DO be respectful of your Instructor.

#4.DO study your nursing plan the night before.

#5. DON'T be late for your clinical

#6. DO be courteous to clinical site staff and classmates.

#7. DON'T make excuses.

#8.DO treat hospital and nursing home equipment with care.

#9.DO follow clinical sites rules as well as Instructors directions.

#10. DON'T drift away from class participation, remember that most learning is in setting.

POW WOW

After the first orientation the Instructors meet once and sometimes twice a week as a group. They work together on lesson plans and development in assuring that the classes are up to the standards set for the nursing program. They also meet on what some would think are the most helpful aspects of the program. Together they identify the more at risk students and mutually search for ways to help and enhance their standing in the program. That way they are able to make and build on suggestions to avoid any students failure in the program. If, however they as a group come to the conclusion that it is best for the student at the time to redirect their energy elsewhere. They will alert this student to other actions needed to continue in the program at another time or transfer to another program that would help them should they want to return to the nursing program.

CLINICAL SITES AT TEACHING HOSPITALS AND NURSING HOMES

Your nursing clinicals will be held at various care centers, nursing homes and hospitals. These facilities have contracts with your nursing school to provide teaching space and patients for you and your fellow students. The patients they provide are a cross section of their hospitalized population or if a nursing home a sample of the less acute residents. These patients are chosen to ensure that you have the opportunity to train at the practice level of the general diseases, illnesses, symptoms and disabilities prevalent in the community today.

You will be assigned one, two to three and maybe four patients depending on how advanced you are at the time.

Reading their charts and discussing them with your Instructor to you knowledge base of said patients. Learning about these patients in this manner will assure you that they are receiving the proper care and medication prescribed for them by the supervisory personnel. You will also be dispensing medication through oral form and through injections and I.V.'s (more on this later). You will be working side by side with on site staff assuring that your patients get to and from their appointments on schedule(this too is important and this too will come up again in our talk).

WORKING WITH CNA'S DURNING YOUR CLINICALS

CNA's (certified nursing assistants) are very, very necessary, in fact, you as a nursing student should have been working as one at sometime, it's part of your necessary training. As mentioned before CNA's deserve our respect they are a part of your team and you are the team leader. Working within your program you receive your report at the beginning of the shift on your patient from your Instructors or the nurses on the prior shift. If your CNA's don't attend this report it is your responsibility to pass on this report to your team members which would include your CNA's. As the team leader it is your job to coordinate your day with your team members. The CNA's may not be aware of the whole picture therefore your job with your team is to supervise as well as attend to your designated duties. You are to show leadership as you supervise your team. You cannot relax and be one of them, you cannot be their peer. On the job you are a supervisor not a friend but you can be friendly and supportive. You cannot be a friend but you can lead by example and firmness tempered with respect for their dignity.

WORKING WITH YOUR PATIENTS IN CLINICALS

On beginning your clinicals you will be asked (as is customary) to introduce yourself to your patients after you have made an assessment of their chart. Once you have an idea of what their illnesses and liabilities are and what medications you will be giving them along with the time. Your nursing Instructor will tell you what she expects you to do and how she/he expects you to conduct your clinical. Such as the forms and charting and physical assessment she wants you to make on your patients.

MEDICATIONS

As a nursing student you will be allowed to dispense medication and you are to be attentive to this. Your Instructor will be evaluating you on this, oral medication is to be given to the patient and you watch as they take it. Some patients will ask you to leave it at their bedside. This is not to be done as this is important to their health and patients have been known to forget it was there, throw it out or just refuse to take it. There is nothing sadder then finding medication left at the bedside or in the bed when moving a patient. There is nothing less satisfying then seeing a patient fail to thrive and finding out they haven't been taking their medication. A nurse can also be penalized for allowing such actions to occur, instructors don't feel that they need to overlook that in their students, it shows that the student is too preoccupied or just doesn't care.

PHYSICAL ASSESSMENTS

On making physical assessments on your patients you will finally get to put into practice everything studied in skills class. The times you practiced on each other are now transformed into using your new found knowledge on your patients. You will now do a complete physical assessment including temperatures, rectal and orals, weights, percussions (if able, it takes practice) of sounds. With heart, lungs, by sight and numerous interview questions on their health problems. Not only are health questions asked but interest is shown in their background, habits and lifestyle changes, those made and those only contemplated. Bring their hearing into consideration, they may or may not be able to hear you.

MAKING ROUNDS AND PRIVACY OF PATIENTS

Being a practicing nursing student you will be asked to make rounds checking on your patients or you accompany your Instructor on such rounds. On these rounds there are patient privacy issues you must respect. You must respect the dignity and privacy of the patient as they are interpreted through their cultural norms. These affect the outcome of your interventions with the patients. When focusing on patient privacy issues during procedures and assessments there are eleven points to practice.

#1. When entering patient's room for procedural or assessment reasons knock on door and wait for permission to enter if need be then close door.

#2. Introduce your self and rest of staff to patient and what they will be doing.

#3. Draw blinds and close privacy curtains especially if patients room is double occupancy.

#4. Drape patient appropriately and use gown if necessary.

#5. Offer patient blanket to avoid chill.

#6. If you are male bring female chaperone when needed if patient is female.

#7. Keep number of people in room to a minimum.

#8. Keep patient informed on procedures to be performed.

#9. Ask patient for permission if more people are needed for observation.

#10. Seek to answer any questions the patient might ask.

WORKING WITH ON SITE NURSES

Doing your clinicals at your rotation sites with nurses who already work there can be a boost to your rotation. The nurses at your clinical site can be wonderful; they want you to succeed there. Many of them still remember how it was when they were students and they want to be helpful to you. Even though most nurses have positive feelings they must be allowed to do their work. Your resource person for your educational nursing questions is your Instructor unless an onsite nurse is assign to you for any type of orientation. Your Instructor follows her lesson plan where as a site nurses way of doing things may differ.

WHAT TIME IS THEIR APPOINTMENT?

On occasions as a student you will be asked to escort your patient to an appointment. It may be out of the facility or it may be to another floor and they might travel in a wheelchair or on a stretcher. Either way once they reach their destination you will be asked to give a verbal report. You must know specific information on how this patient might react to certain stimulation or if diabetic when was the last time they had their insulin. Can they walk, how do they transfer out of wheelchair or into wheelchair, do they speak and are they hard of hearing. Perhaps they are anxious or afraid; this must be communicated to the healthcare professional receiving them. One way or the other you will have to be knowledgeable about your patient.

WHAT IS AN EVAL

An eval is your evaluation on your nursing abilities to be performed by your nursing Instructor. This is when your Instructor calls you into his/her office to give you the good/bad news of how well you are doing in your class work. A good or bad evaluation can inspire or mentally depress you, these are usually done in the middle of each class rotation while you are in nursing school. If doing badly in class you can be dropped from the program. Once you graduate and assume your job duties as a working nurse you are entitled to your evaluation in person from your nursing supervisor at least once a year. This is used to alert you to any problems you may have on the job and when and if you deserve a raise.

YOUR LIBRARY, LOVE IT

Studying in the library is great; you have literally hundreds and thousands of books to assist you in your endeavors. It has comfortable chairs and the quiet is in abundance so absorb it at your own pace. First thing to do is find a good spot off to the side out of traffic where you will interrupt no one and no one will interrupt you. If you like facing the door then find a seat facing the door. This is one of the few places where speaking loudly or making noise is frowned upon so you shouldn't be disturbed. This noiseless atmosphere should help you to put in anywhere from one and one half to two hours studying at one time. If you happen to be operating on more study time then sleep and you don't have any other place to go. Then you are in the right place, the library is also an excellent place to take a power nap. Make it a deep sleep and don't worry, the Librarian is watching over you.

Your reading and studying should follow a schedule, one that you are able to adjust and adapt to any situation. When you are ready to study choose the subject and set a reasonable time limit to study. Have everything you need to complete this session and prioritize the important things. Show yourself kindness, treat yourself as a guest and chart your progress realistically. By all means take your breaks, go for a short walk and talk to friends. Read an interesting magazine or the daily newspaper. It's healthy to distract your mind occasionally and it beneficial to your memory. If need be, mentally convert it into a game that you are intent on winning, have fun with your studies.

EXAMS

"The sum of your knowledge shall be revealed through the performance of your actions." A wise man said that but I don't think he had nursing exams in mind. All of the studying and quizzes are dedicated to one thing, assuring that you pass your final exam in the NCLEX-RN or the NCLEX-PN. It's true that your Instructors use and, reuse questions from the NCLEX's, they are just revised and reformulated for your pleasure. Served especially for you in different wordings but meaning the same thing. There are only so many ways a question can be posed to you asking. "What is the pathophysiology of infectious/inflammatory renal and urologic problems? The answer to that question will be the same no matter how many different ways the question is asked. There can theoretically be ten different NCLEX books but logically and numerically that same question can be asked only three different ways before the so-called average person can recognize the pattern. Hence, reading the assignment in the book two times and supplementing that with studying the questions on the pathophysiology of infectious/ inflammatory Renal and urologic problems in three to four different NCLEX's will serve to cut your studying in half and prepare you for that exam be it weekly exams or finals.

WHICH IS IT LPN/LVN OR RN

Which do you want to be an LPN/LVN or an RN? Either way joining the nursing profession is a big stept in the right direction in service to humanity. In the beginning the two programs were separate, you either enrolled into the LPN/LVN program or the RN program. Now for the sake of simplicity or otherwise the two programs in some cases have merged. Offering the student the choice of ending their studies at LPN/LVN and graduating or continuing on into the RN program and graduating. The RN program by its very length and depth is more complicated offering much more substantial courses.

Due to the inherent shortage of RN's the LPN/LVN program has been forced to fill some areas left vacant by the absence of RN's. The charge nurse slot was traditionally filled by RN's but of late some of those jobs have been filled by LPN/LVN's.

Until the RN population is able to increase LPN/LVN's will have to increase their educational opportunities to fill in leaving RN's free for supervision.

PROTECTING YOUR BACK

Nursing is built on moving patients, moving them from bed to bath and to chair and to other places in between. You need to turn and roll them, walk them and at times carry them. Some patients are weaker than at other times and can get sicker or are your patient because they are unable to get from point A to point B by themselves. When untrained or trained for that matter in transporting patients physically, the back is the prime target for a breakdown. We suffer from backaches, slipped disks, pinched nerves and other ailments all from unsafe and multiple lifting. You will be trained in the safe art of lifting and pivoting patients along with the large array of lifting machines available to nursing personal.

CLINICAL TRADITION

You might think I'm jumping ahead of myself by mentioning this but there is a clinical tradition I love to perpetuate. If anyone has an unsuccessful rotation at their clinical site they won't be around to notice. This is for those of you who have a totally successful clinical rotation. You're happy, very happy and believe it or not your hosting clinical site nurses are happy for you. Tradition states that the nursing students get together and buy treats for the staff on their ward. Nothing elaborate just donuts and coffee cake, anything that will bring a smile.

MEDICAL TERMS OR FOREIGN LANGUAGE

Lets face it medical terminology is a strange, wonderful foreign and ancient language. It's all rooted in Latin and gobbedligook, just try to say exacerbation three times fast. See what I mean, you not only need to know what these terms mean but you need to know how to pronounce them. You need this knowledge and you need it as soon as you start in nursing school. There are classes offered during nursing classes or prior. Your medical Terminology class will be helpful for you to recognize your medications, diseases, muscle parts and it might also come in handy in pronouncing some doctors names.

TEN THINGS YOU NEED TO BECOME A GOOD NURSE

#1. A strong back: Most care centers are now calling themselves a no lift facility ... Don't believe it, you have to move patients, help them move or prevent them from falling and believe me your back will come into play.

#2.Patience: You will need the patience of a mother and then some. While being a mom would entitle you the privilege of sometimes speaking to your children in a raised voice. Being a nursing student/nurse you have no such outlets, if you did, that would fall into the status of patient abuse. That (depending on the severity) would make you subject to disciplinary action against you up to and including discharge from the program.

#3.Math aptitude: Medication is dispensed through measurements, mg, ml, oz, etc. The nurse must be familiar with these while reading medication orders notes

#4. Memory: At times the nursing student will be caring for several patients (one, two or three) and the nurse must be able to mentally differentiate between and keep their orders separate in mind.

#5. Diplomatic: At times the nursing student/nurse will be sought to take sides among different factions she/

he supervises. Except under extenuating circumstances the nurse should remain neutral.

#6. Endurance: Due to the unforeseeable circumstances of the medical profession, a nurse must be able to work past established meal times and self toileting schedules. Meaning there is not always time to have lunch or heed the call of nature. When a patient becomes suddenly incapacitated or ill everything else has to wait.

#7. Reliability: Staff and facility need to know that when needed the nurse will cover the areas assigned to her/him.

#8. Protocol: Adhere to such protocol in following the orders of Doctors/Nurse practitioners and other superiors as prescribed by facility.

#10. Leadership: Practice leadership and utilize that and capable qualities in junior staff members.

NOTES PAGE 1

NOTES PAGE 2

NOTES PAGE 3

NOTES PAGE 4

NOTES PAGE 5

NOTES PAGE 6

NOTES PAGE 7

NOTES PAGE 8

NOTES PAGE 9

NOTES PAGE 10

COMFORTS OF HOME

Full time nursing school is intensive at times and at other times it's a waiting game. Providing you don't have to rush home after a morning class, you may have your classes spread out over the whole day. Your classes may be so scheduled that you literally have to be at school eight to twelve hours for three maybe four or less classes a day. When not using down time studying you could spend it in the student lounge watching TV. You might also want to utilize the free time afforded by the school gym. There is also the study lab or computer room as well as places to watch movies. If a shower and change of clothing is needed, the locker room of the gym is just the place.

SECURITY

Most nursing schools, colleges, etc. employ their own security safeguarding students as well as their belongings. In some schools shuttle cabs are available to students if needed to get to and from any distant parking. School lockers for coats and books are generally accessible throughout the buildings near the classrooms. Should you be unable to open your locker or lose your key, security is nearby to open it for you.

BREAKS AND LUNCH

In nursing school you may get an hour for lunch now but in clinicals if you are doing a full shift you are entitled to a half hour for lunch and possibly a fifteen minute break. Your Instructor would expect you to conform to this schedule whether you want to or not. The best advice you can get is to follow the rules and advice your Instructor lays out for you. Once you graduate the rules aren't as clear cut along those matters. While as a new nurse you may find yourself in the middle of a treatment or in an emergency situation that demands your full attention and effort. When lunch time rolls around, you can't just up and say "Oh, its lunch time ta-ta." Continuity is needed in health care. As noted before there are days all too often when seriously speaking you won't even have time go to lunch.

CONFIDENTIALITY

What does confidentially mean to a nursing student? It means that by not betraying the confidence of your patients such as giving out private information to unauthorized persons. Leaving any forms or other paperwork such as social security numbers unsecured and out in the open or discussing patients anywhere you can be overheard. You are leaving yourself open to legal action as well as discipline as a student or termination of your employment if you are found to violate the rules of confidentially when you begin your career as a nurse.

REFUSAL OF MEDS

As a rule when you're a nursing student your clinical site prefers to have you assigned to patients who are compliant. Meaning they are very cooperative with the nursing staff. Enjoy it because when you graduate all the kid gloves will come off. You will begin your dispensing of meds to a few of your patients who will not be so compliant. There will be various ways and reasons of refusing medication oral or otherwise. Some oral meds will be refused with a curt "no," just remember patients have their rights and we will go more into that later. They have a right to say no and some will punctuate that with a punch or shove and seasoned with a few swear words. Most of the patients want to be helped but not all of them are responsible for their actions. If you feel you need to be persistent do so with caution.

UNMANAGEABLE PATIENTS IN YOUR ROTATION

As I said earlier during your rotation, your clinical site, your nursing school and your Instructor want you to be safe. Not just with your patients but for yourself as well. However on occasions there may be a mix-up or miss assignment leaving you and your patient at risk. They may assign you a stressed out or violent patient, just to be on the safe side treat your patient as your Instructor directs you. Be efficient and respectful as you would all of your patients.

PATIENT ABUSE

Patient abuse can take many forms, some of those obvious; some are subtle and can be under your radar. Handling a patient roughly physically is one of the more obvious abuses but did you know that just telling a patient that you are short on staff is also patient abuse. So it's not just the physical abuse we are on the alert for but it's the psychological aspects we want to curtail. Abuse takes many forms. If a staff member is seen committing patient abuse and you say nothing to your superiors about it, you are just as guilty as the person who committed it and the punishment has been known to be severe.

FAMILY MEMBERS

In nursing the student nurses are taught that not only is the patient treated but the family is also factored in to the treatment. The family affects the health of the patient and influences how the patient reacts to the nurses' efforts and vice-versa. Students are taught not to ignore family members and listen to their concerns and questions. Treated with respect by staff you will find that the family is a valuable resource for the student nurse. Another point to remember is that the family has a source of valuable information and usually have significant influence over the patient.

STAFF ABUSE

Of course we've touched this segment of abuse. After leaving nursing school hopefully not during, all of your patients won't be the ones you've dreamed about. You remember those that are eternally grateful for your care and professionalism. Your patients can run the length of the spectrum from the kindly little old lady who reminds you of your sweet grandmother. To, if you're lucky, the big burly gentleman the police bring in wearing handcuffs and leg irons for you to treat for gunshot wounds. Don't worry, they usually send a few police officers to protect you. You need not worry about that either, you have a better chance of winning the big lottery statically speaking.

Some patients in long term care are habitually violent to staff, hopefully their medication has been readjusted for that. Some strike out when they feel that staff aggressively invades their space. Others can be maladjusted, having little or no impulse control. The little guy in their head may tell them to strike out at you and there is no gatekeeper to prevent this although psychiatry is coming a long ways towards addressing this issue.

It is up to you to be vigilant when confronted with this type of patient but at the same time you don't wish to bring harm to the patient. You will be taught ways of defusing the different situations you may come into contact with. When professional fighters converge in their big bout the referee issues his last words to them. This is good advice for nursing students/nurses as well. "Protect yourself at all times."

SEXUAL HARASSMENT

One thing the public frowns on especially since the confirmation of a certain Supreme Court Justice a few years ago. It's one more thing student nurses are getting a full sermon about from their nursing Instructors, Sexual Harassment. In nursing school and throughout your working career you will be caring for some patients who are suffering from dementia and those who have no such excuse. Some of those will be sexually aggressive patients (maybe some coworkers) who can't keep their hands to themselves. The demented patients are not entirely responsible for their actions; however the others can be a handful. The patients suffering from this dementia can be helped by some medications but you have to help by charting and reporting such behaviors. You can also help yourself and others by forming a team of two with your coworkers when entering their rooms and taking a firm business like attitude and not giving them the idea that you might be flirting. The operative word when caring for patients of this type is assertiveness.

DIFFICULT CLASSMATES OR COWORKERS

At some time you may come across classmates whom you would classify as difficult to work with or even to be around. Don't wait long enough to make each other miserable to the point where it may affect your work. Make attempts to settle your differences together. This would be your practice to prepare for your nursing career where given the odds you will ultimately meet a coworker who will bring the same displeasure out in you. Explore using conflict resolution to end your disagreements.

THAT SMALL BUT EFFICIENT MINORITY MALE NURSE

Male nurses are pioneers, like women are when they decide that they won't be regulated to what small minded people denote as women's jobs. More men are becoming nurses and by the same percentage more women are becoming doctors. Men have proven that they are just as efficient as women in the nurses' role. Established female nurses and those turning to instruction have encouraged the entry of male nurses as well as female nurses.

QUESTION: AS A MAN, NURSING STUDENT OR WORKING NURSE, WHAT SINGLE INCIDENT GAVE YOU PAUSE ON ENTERING NURSING?

ANSWER:

#1. I learned to look at female nurses in general from a different point of view, they didn't look at me as just a man, they treated me as an equal.

#2. One woman outright called me a pervert because as a nurse I would see female patients in the nude.

#3. As a working nurse two different patients husbands refuse to let me care for their wives because as a black man I would see them unclothed.

#4. Believe it or not we men are welcome where I work because we are always asked to lift heavy objects.

#5. One female volunteer at the facility where I work vocally objected to me toileting a female patient whom I had been caring for during the last five years because I'm a man.

#6. Some people find it easier to believe that the man is the patient rather then the nurse.

This short questionnaire in no way suggests that men have it harder then women in any professional endeavors. It just states the point of view of six men both student nurses and established working nurses.

PATIENTS RIGHTS

Congress in answer to past inequities in the health care system passed what is called the Patients Bill of Rights. This bill is to guarantee patients a say in their health care. Some people may not agree with its guidelines but the medical community has a duty to follow the law to this respect. You need to know that outside of extreme circumstances your patients have a right to refuse their medication at anytime. They also have the right to refuse any treatments they don't want and to speak with their doctor if able. When you are working as a student nurse dispensing medication you are required or asked by certain facilities to inform the patient of any consequences there may be in not taking medication as prescribed. Patient education is a vital role of the nurse. Refusal of treatment requires documentation that the patient made an informed decision. That means, the patient is aware of any risks or benefits prior to making their decision.

PLAYING FAVORITES

As a nursing student you may be tempted but you are to be discouraged from showing favoritism when caring for two or more patients where it can be seen. Jealousy is a natural emotion as we are dealing with human beings who could be vying for the nurse's attention. We should expect jealousy as a by-product to be seen when two patients feel they each have developed a special bond with a nurse and the nurse appears to enjoy spending more time with another patient or just showing them more attention. It could be argued that some patients are more likeable then others.

However, we as professionals need to stay within our boundaries to accomplish our task. When it appears that we are playing one patient against another we should expect conflict and to avoid this we need to be professional. Our patients depend on us and we need to show impartiality concerning their mental as well as their physical health.

NURSES BURN OUT

Do nurses burn out? I would say yes, just as much burnout as anyone else in any other job that literally balances life and death. When health care facilities assign work with no regards of if it can be done safely or even in a timely manner that can add stress to the nurse carrying that assignment. When the staff needed to care for a certain number of patients is cut in half and expected to do the same job in the same amount of time I would say that contributes to burnout. When the health and very lives of patients depend on certain equipment and its not available or even works properly that adds to burnout. When staff nurses are forced to work more hours then they can or want to then job fatigue follows. Those reasons are why we so desperately need new competent nurses and if you are willing to study for all of the right reasons then you can be a nurse.

SMOKING

Right now care facilities are working hard in the movement to obliterate smoking. It is gradually being phased out of existence due to the new regulations being passed not only by the care facilities themselves but by our lawmakers. Smoking causes countless health problems and aggravates many others yet an enormous number of people continue such practices. To see a nurse or any other health professional indulge goes against the very nature of their profession.

Right now health care centers are in a race with time to ban smoking in and around their campuses. Some of the more progressive care centers are banning it even from their parking lot. Neither staff nor visitors are allowed to even smoke in their cars while they are parked on facility lots.

The local, state and federal government is competing in their own race to see who can collect the most lucrative taxes on cigarettes. As one of the most visible health professions now is the time for the new crop of nurses to set the example.

BI LINGUAL

The United States has always been blessed with its diversity in population, we as its citizens have at our disposal all of the living languages of the world. We are even able to communicate in some of the so-called dead languages that are no longer in widespread use. Never has the nursing profession been in more need of bi-lingual nurses to interpret the concerns of the health care community to the patients and back to the nursing care givers. They are not only needed in nursing homes and hospitals but in our schools, public and private. Our communities specifically asked for them and health care should be accessible to all of our citizens. Should you as a bi-lingual nursing student be interested the nursing profession would be proud to put your language abilities to use in the health care system.

MRSA

Have you ever wondered why nursing students and the medical community at large are required to wash their hands so often? Well, it's the same reason your mother always told you to wash your hands before you came to dinner. Its germs, the same germs that can be passed from one person to another and in succession can make us all sick. There are millions of germs and just as many different types. Some are beneficial to us (the good ones) and some of them are at the opposite end of the spectrum (the bad ones), they can make us all very ill and cause infections that can kill. I want to make notice of a particular germ. MRSA is Methicillin-Resistant Staphylococcus Aureus, this is a super bacteria. It is resistant to common antibiotics, causing infections that can't easily be cured and it can be passed on to others like any other bacteria. It can be passed on to you and other patients and even your own family if strict hand washing is not practiced. You as a nursing student must join in and enforce the hand washing rule and learn more about MRSA in your studies.

EXAM GLOVES

What was formally known as just rubber gloves used in the hospitals has expanded to be label as exam gloves. There are many types, there is latex, flex vinyl, powder free, nitrile powder-free, sterile and non sterile gloves. Latex is rarely used because of the allergy it causes many people.

Some people in the medical community have found that different types of gloves have literally become a health hazard to them. For some it's a little matter of trial and error in finding which gloves they can tolerate. With some gloves such as latex the body reacts with a rash or hives or worse anaphylactic shock, a medical and potentially fatal emergency. Some care workers have been known to lose tolerances over time which has sadly caused them to abandon their profession in a search of relief from the allergic reaction they cause them. Others find that they can keep rashes under control with hand lotions and other products. That what must be mentioned is that hand washing and gloves compliment each other. Some gloves can be porous and bacteria may be able to pass through gloves going either way.

NOTES AND CHARTING

Notes and charting provide for the continuity of nursing and health care. It literally allows for someone to continue the safe and effective health care you are providing your patients. It is the essential communication between health care givers and those of the supervisory personnel. There are different types of note making and charting on your patients you will be asked to do. The type that your Instructor prefers is most likely what you will be doing in nursing school. While this manual does not profess to be an instruction book on charting it is only to alert you to what you will be expected to do. The charting must be concise, to the point and hopefully legible. When hand writing notes in patient records there must no white out and no continuous crossing out of words to make it unreadable. When striking out a word one line through it is suffice and written over the word should be written the word void. Medical charting is considered a legal document and could be a legal document although not discounted by all medical personal, this author strongly urges you to not chart other staff members names. Only mention nurse, CNA or any other title if needed.

MED ERRORS

A med error is something like a curse that I wouldn't wish on anyone. Why? Because it's the patient who suffers, not usually the staff member who dispenses the medication although if habitually done can lead to repercussions. There is a rule about giving out medication; it's called the five rights. Right med, right patient, right time, right dose and right route. Since this manual in no way pretends to be a medical text book, I will leave the rest up to your independent reading and your Instructor to explore this more in depth.

Always remember giving the wrong dose to the wrong patient is a no-no. If need be read and re-read your medication orders to be sure. When you begin to give out your medication your Instructor will supervise you until she/he considers you competent. Don't be in a hurry, read and comprehend your medication orders, you only have one chance to give a medication correctly.

READING THE CHARTS

This may be one of the most difficult things you will ever have to do in your life and that is trying to read other peoples handwriting. When handwritten charting is done it is usually done while the person is in a hurry. Whether it is written so fast because of a lack of time and or just because it is habitually done. Whichever it is it is still difficult to read for the regular chart reader and even more so for the nursing student/beginner. T's look like O's and A's look like whatever. When attempting to gain information from the chart, your imagination can run amok as a new reader. You can start to sweat and you mutter maybe under your breath or out loud "Please God what have they written?"

It's been jokingly said that doctors use chicken scratches when they write, well they aren't' the only ones. Penmanship isn't as revered as much as it used to be. When you regularly start to handwrite what seems like a million notes you too will scrimp on words and letters. Just remember to think kind thoughts of the person who will have to read them behind you. If you find you don't know if you are looking at a chart upside down or sideways, ask your colleague what that word looks like. Sometimes all you need is a new perspective from a different point of view in life. Fortunately more and more facilities are using computerized charting.

NURSES BEFORE US

Nurses were once thought of as non professionals, they were invisible to the naked eye unless you were hospitalized. They were thought more as a combination of the maid and servants of the doctors. Nurses began as the volunteers of the conscience, watching the suffering and seeking to alleviate it. In the very beginning nurses were not paid at all, they were the ones who collected money and supplies from charitable donations and used it to help those in need.

Nursing was dominated by a certain type of woman, those that felt the need to help the less fortunate. If a person was looking to get rich none of them looked toward nursing. Some women and unfortunately a few nurses thought of it as an occupation to mark time until they were able to get married. As the years went by at the very least nurses commanded low pay and even less respect. No one really knew or cared that nurses were emerging as highly trained and performing their various duties at a high level of proficiency. The stories that follow the lifeline of nursing are numerous and exciting. They are encouraging and informative as well as thought provoking.

Nursing today has become more and more specialized just as other professions thus it is producing more and more burnout. It could be a correction in the profession eliminating those who can't change with the future or it could be through the mismanagement of those at the top. Either way nursing is and will continue fulfilling its destiny as a cornerstone of the medical profession. Each nurse working today and those to come, like any other profession, owes a great debt of gratitude to those who came before them. Taking this space to spotlight two individuals out of the millions of past nurses and to present their stories is my privilege. Before I do I want to state that no two stories are the same just as no two nurses are the same. These are the stories of two different nurses, two of the nurses who came before us. Two who are as different as can be although they were united in the same profession. They shared the same dreams of becoming nurses and they became nurses coming from two different directions. Ultimately they met and became fast friends.

DOLORES

The idea of becoming a nurse was obviously born along with Dolores as some people said. Her first view of the world was the Wisconsin farm her parents owned outside of the small town of Denmark. Growing up an only child left her with a lot of free time which she began to put to good use as she helped her parents on the farm. Doing what all children on a farm will do , helping to milk cows, feeding chickens and collecting eggs, many of those animals she thought of as her personal pets. Her morning chores were done before walking to school and assisting her teacher in getting the classroom ready before the other students arrived

She secretly nurtured the dream of becoming a nurse after an aunt was forced through the unkind circumstances of becoming ill, to move into the family living room to recover. An enterprising eight year old Dolores soon fashioned an exact replica of a nurse's hat out of paper to help care for her.

When not doing her farm chores she continued her memberships to the various clubs that were available in school during the years of World War II, such as the 4H club, collecting metal and cloth for the war effort. Volunteering as a secretary for the music club offered her the chance of assisting classmates in expressing their love for music in her junior and senior years of high school.

Showing independence not normally celebrated in a young woman of her generation. She rejected any money offered by her parents to pay for nursing school, opting to earn it herself. Shortly after graduation from high school she began her full time working career. At the age of eighteen she worked as a nurses helper, gathering valuable experience from the health care field.

Noted for her caring disposition by friends and family she was soon sought out to help with and care for the children of these and members of her church.

Doing this she soon felt she had earned enough money to begin her studies. Not long after applying she was accepted to the Mt. Sinai School of Nursing, a chance to enter into the career she dreamed of. She happily and excitedly moved to Milwaukee to enroll in their program in what was to be a life of structured dormitory life. The world of a nursing student proved to be a rigorous life. A nursing student's life that she was able to successfully navigate in her first journey away from the watchful eyes of her mother.

Attending a chaperoned outing and meeting a special young man was all "the rage" at that time. Dolores was no different than any of the other young women in the dorm, she met her special guy at just such an outing. Love was not too far away however nursing school took precedent, the love of nursing was much stronger at the time. Nursing classes and the years seem to rush by, she had the two great loves of her life and she though it would never end.

Graduation brought with it the title RN and her parents came to Milwaukee to celebrate her passage and new challenges, as well as a new job to go with her maturing relationship. Not long after graduation she had another special day, she married her special young man and went to work at West Allis Memorial Hospital.

After the appropriate time, given they were newlyweds they were blessed with a beautiful baby girl. Still eager to continue her career she quietly returned to work gaining the reputation among her peers as a tireless no nonsense staff nurse. Along with advancing her career she was also advancing her family, 17 months later another beautiful baby girl. Not wanting to be away from her young children she took a temporary mothers retirement to be at home with her girls. In a span of years she would give birth to two more children a boy and a girl to add to her brood before she would return to work. Working the third shift at the hospital during 14 years she included 4 more beautiful tiny ones to round out the family, sadly one baby girl not surviving. Marking her 25 years at the hospital she retired.

LILLIE

Lillie's life began similarly to Dolores's as her first view of the world was also of a farm her parents worked. She was one of fourteen children that blessed her parents in the state of Arkansas in the late 20's. Although she was neither the oldest nor the youngest her siblings still looked to Lillie for words of encouragement in their young lives. While still a child she would be the busy-body around the house, she was mother's little helper with her younger sisters and brothers. Even while helping to work the farm at such a young age she still found time to keep up with her school studies.

Growing up normally then would be called growing up fast now; the teen years were an intro to middle age. She became a typical young teenage bride in a marriage that produced three strapping boys and a beautiful tiny baby girl.

Nothing lasts forever and a marriage vow made by a young girl can be dissolved by a mature woman. Especially when she starts to make decisions for her children as well as herself. Moving to another city and vowing to make a new life for herself and her children she started over. Not much later she finally met her prince in this strange new city. She looked love in the eye and she married him, a union that was to last 56 years. Along with her new husband came his beautiful young daughter which made for a splendid blended family.

Together they moved to a city on a lake, Milwaukee, Wisconsin where her future in the health care field began and during this time they were joined by the arrival of a final lovely daughter. It was sometime before then that she began her job as a health care worker. A Job that very few people wanted at the time, a job that would even horrify certain people.

She became an Attendant, what today would be called a Nurses aid. She worked on the old Milwaukee County grounds at the Muirdale Tuberculosis Sanatorium. A facility in the 1940's through the early 1960's that was set apart from the other health care service buildings due to its functions. It served as a depository for Tuberculosis patients. A disease that never failed to claimed as victims some of its own health care staff. Many times she was tested as having come into contact With TB. Due to the close proximity of staff and patients many care workers were retired due to contracting the disease.

On the closing of the facility Lillie moved on to the County Hospital and there with the encouragement from coworkers, friends and family made her decision to continue her education and become a nurse. Enrolling into the Milwaukee Area Technical college to begin her studies. From there she transferred to the UWM Milwaukee nursing school and in 1979 she graduated as an RN. Completing her journey as a nurse with the Milwaukee County health care system in 1987 she retired.

LILLIE AND DOLORES

They had so much in common, yet that one Saturday would be the first time that they would actually meet. Their introductions to each other carried even more significance at the time as both were retired nurses.

More so even at the wedding, while one was the mother of the bride and the other was the mother of the groom. Lillie's son was a nurse and Dolores's daughter was also a nurse, each one inevitably inspired by the life's career choice of their respective parent. On those points alone they had long conversations which lasted well into the evening. They spoke of the idiosyncrasies of the doctors and the always formidability of the charge nurse. Laughing at such silliness, they readily admitted to being such a charge nurse.

As the night wore on they eagerly traded phone numbers and they both promised to meet again at what was supposed to be the beginnings of new combined family functions. The next new family function never came as Lillie and her husband Buddy began to make plans to spend their retirement years in Las Vegas, Nevada.

Settling down to continue her own retirement Dolores made it a point to enjoy her children and grandchildren's company along with that of her in laws and that special son-in-law of hers who showed promise as a nurse.

Two years later Dolores was told by her daughter that Lillie was returning for a visit. Thinking it would be fun to discuss nursing and retirement with her friend and counterpart Dolores made plans for a small shopping foray just the two of them.

Meeting Lillie again Dolores knew she was different, with her familiar smile, there was no secret knowing that nurses shared with each other. Lillie did not recognize her, being the retired nurse she didn't need her daughter to tell her that Lillie was suffering from Alzheimer's.

EPILOG

...Lillie and Dolores went on that shopping spree anyway accompanied by their son and daughter, the now old married couple. Dolores trudging along with her walker (supporting a painful hip) holding Lillie's hand and guiding her to the different racks of clothes they both knew they would never buy. Lillie returned to Las Vegas with Buddy where she died of a sudden stroke three years later.

SO, YOU WANT TO BE A NURSE

Nursing students come from all walks of life; they represent all faiths and cultures. Some will have more obstacles to overcome than others but they all will exhibit the same dedication to achieving their goals. In the challenges you will meet in your education you will show the same commendable effort as those that came before you. Your success will inspire the efforts of those who will come after you. Good luck in your studies and your career as a nurse!

To contact the author go to wjfloater@msn.com

NURSING

BY

BEATRICE BAKER MED, MSN, R.N.

To those individuals who want to become nurses. Everyone has heard about the nursing shortage and how it has affected the healthcare industry. The nurse shortage is real and although you may not be hearing about it as often as you have in previous years, you can be assured it still exists. There is a lack of skilled nursing staff to take care of the patient in hospitals and clinics. This lack of skilled personnel has led to the increase in less skilled professionals (i.e. nurse aides or nurse technicians) assuming the duties and responsibilities previously held bt the registered nurse (RN). The nurse shortage has also become a reason for nursing schools to increase enrollment for certified nurse's aides to return to school and become Professional Nurses.

You may be one of those individuals who want to become a Registered Nurse or you my know someone who in planning on becoming an R.N. and entering the nursing profession. For all those prospective nurses who have decided they want to become nurses, I say to you that you are about to embark on a wonderful career. Before entering into nursing school there are several things you should look at. First, request literature from at least three of the nursing schools you might want to attend. Second, compare the schools, looking at such information as is the school accredited, how many students does the school graduate each year and how many students per year pass the state board examination. Third, check to see which school will offer tutoring and counseling as part of their program. The fourth thing to look for before making your choice is where are most of the graduates working, what hospitals or what area of nursing.

If most nursing students take time to visit several schools and check to see if the school graduates are doing well in their chosen profession they will be able to make an informed and wise choice for their educational goals. When students choose a nursing school that is capable of teaching them using adult principles along with using the latest advances in technology they are more likely to be successful in their new chosen profession.